I0439890

Increase Your Libido

Proven methods for permanently increasing your libido, sex drive, and sexual confidence

(The ultimate guide to always being in the mood)

Table of Contents

Introduction

I want to thank you as well as congratulate you for downloading the book, *"Increase Your Libido"*.

The pace of everyday life, stress, and fatigue often undermine your sexual desire. The lack of libido does not only cloud your relationship with your partner, but also affects your general well being. Learn how to increase libido with natural techniques and stimulants in order to enjoy your sexuality once again.

Libido is the vital energy that keeps us connected with desire and sexuality. The decrease or lack of libido can affect you physically and emotionally. It can cause problems with your partner, too. They may misinterpret your lack of desire for something else.

The food aphrodisiacs often are the first to be invoked, when increasing libido. However, these are not the only answer. There are many ways to fix your libido, which includes foods, exercises, physician consultation, and even natural aphrodisiacs to stimulate the senses. They may not be a part of your daily diet, but you can use them as a valuable supplement to boost your sexual desire.

This book will not only give you the Holy Grail to increasing your libido, but it will also give you a few tips which you did not know about heightening your libido. So, please, sit back, relax, and enjoy your read. It's definitely going to be worth your time.

Chapter 1: Reason of Sexual Desire

It happens to almost all couples with the passage of time; your partner has the feeling that his or her desire for sex is higher than that of yours. Such misunderstanding can generate much confusion in a couple's married life. However, it can easily be solved if you know the right techniques.

For a long time, and even today, it has been assumed that men always want to have sex more than women. *This is just not true*. The reality is that, men and women have the same needs from sex, as well as the same desires -though their cycles work quite differently. This has continued to confuse the experts for a long time.

According to a literature review published in the *Canadian Medical Association Journal*, which analyzes a large number of studies that have been conducted since the 90s on female sexual dysfunction, there has been a repeated tendency to identify sexual desire as the initial step that gives women a strong sexual relationship.

According to this view of sex, the absence of this "desire" could be a problem. A dysfunction, according to numerous surveys, may affect around a third of all men and women between 18 and 59 years. But, is it really the absence of a genuine sexual desire or is it something that should be considered normal?

The reality is that according to Dr. Rosemary Basson, researcher at the Center for Sexual Medicine in Vancouver (Canada), and author of the *Revision*, sexual desire does not have to be present so that a woman would want to have sex.

The female libido increases with time. Women reach sexual maturity around age 35, whereas men reach their sexual peak around the age of 25. The desire, however, is affected by the very routine of a relationship. As explained by sexologists Sarah Murray and Robin Milhausen, from the University of Ontario (Canada), in a study published in the journal *Sex & Marital Therapy*, sexual desire in women may weaken as time passes by.

Nonetheless, this does not mean that women no longer want to have sex. They just have different motivations for doing so. In many cases, women seek to foster emotional intimacy with their partner or to increase their self-esteem. Sexual desire, therefore, is not present at the onset of the sexual intercourse, but it appears later on. Men do this as well, except men also seek out sex for pleasure.

This is basically the key to understanding why women do not always seem as responsive as men regarding sexual acts. The good news is that you can work on that sexual desire. With proper stimulation, sexual arousal, and pleasure, sexual desire can be intensified and relationships can become more satisfying.

For Arousing a Woman

The American sexologist, Laurie Watson, provides a number of tips to raise libido in women. These tips can be useful for couples who are looking to increase their sexual frequency.

Make Some Plans

Roberto Sanz, sexologist of Sexpol Foundation, explained in a recent article published in *"The Confidential"* that sex does not need to be always spontaneous. In fact, it is very difficult to achieve it beyond the first few months of dating. So, make a plan about this activity. Make the atmosphere feel sexy along with dinner, round up some great movies, and some other mini-activities. Pornography might just help, too!

Build Up the Heat with Some Foreplay

As Basson notes in his study, a number of women engage in sex without having a true desire. However, if sex goes well, the desire could just develop or emerge. Many men have trouble accepting that there are times when their wives only make love just to please them. There is some truth to that, but not really completely. Sometimes, women just need to warm up a bit. Basically, what can be done to resolve this is to introduce foreplay before the sexual intercourse. Give out some love through cuddling as well as do some little naughty acts here and there to get her excited. Watson further explains that sex may end up being wild and passionate with the inclusion of foreplay. He says that the greater the excitement invoked, the more pleasant the orgasms will be.

Timing is Everything

No matter how much you would want the sex to push through, you still have to consider great timing. Women cannot focus on sex if they have problems of emotional nature. After a fight, for example, it makes no sense to make love. Women tend to take into account a lot of things after a fight and sex would be the last on their list. The best timing is when things are not emotionally burdening to your lady love or when there is something to be celebrated about. When women are happy to start with, they would be able to enjoy sex better.

Orgasm Should Not Always be the Goal

To a man, a satisfying sexual relationship comes with an awesome orgasm, but according to Watson, this is not always the case with women. To women, in many cases, they simply want to experience the pleasures of the intercourse - not only the orgasm. Some men who are not aware of this feel very frustrated. Most men think that for a woman to be satisfied, she must also reach the orgasmic phase. Orgasm is not always the goal for women. Women are in for sex to feel the pleasure and the love their partners have to give.

Chapter 2: Increasing Your Libido

"Libido" is a term that is directly associated with sexual desire. It is often described as the energy or sexual drive felt by individuals. However, a person's libido will not always at its highest peak and there are many reasons why. One of the main reasons for a decreasing libido is poor diet followed by a regular rhythm of inappropriate life. Fortunately, there simple steps that can be followed to help increase libido.

It is recommended that **diets should include, if not based, on the "aphrodisiac foods"**. There is a long list of the so-called "aphrodisiac foods". Some of those on the list would include chocolates, oysters, dairy, lean meat, and poultry products to name a few. These foods contain elements that can help boost libido. One of these elements, for instance, is zinc. Zinc can help in increasing the production of testosterone in men, thereby increasing their libido in the process.

It is also very important to **reduce the excessive consumption of carbohydrates**, especially those rich in sugar because sugar can increase the normal levels of insulin in the blood. Such increase is directly reflected in the production of testosterone decreasing production and causing a decrease in libido.

A good blood circulation can also help in increasing one's libido. Omega 3 is essential for having a good blood circulation throughout the body. A good blood circulation can boost blood in the genitals. Incidentally, Omega 3 also raises dopamine levels in the brain. Dopamine is a major precursor to get in the "mood" since it offers a feel-good feeling.

Always remember that **smoking can also harm one's libido levels**. Not only is smoking harmful to the body in general, but it is also harmful for one's libido since it can greatly reduce sexual pleasure because of its major component - nicotine. Unfortunately, if you smoke regularly, this can build up over time and restrict the arteries. Once the arteries are restricted, proper blood flow will not occur - you know how proper blood circulation is important, right?

When it comes to increasing the libido, the **best results can be achieved with the aid of a good workout**. Regularly working out can help in producing high levels of testosterone in men. Among the best performing exercises we can find the squat or bench press. In addition to that, regular workout will also ensure a proper blood flow and a fit body. Isn't a fit body quite enticing in bed?

Consuming natural supplements like g**inseng and ginkgo biloba or damiana** can also help in improving blood flow while also increasing energy. Both of these are apparently two key factors when it comes to heightening the libido.

A great contribution to enhancing one's libido is **reducing stress**. For these methods such as yoga, deep breathing exercises, meditation, and even regular exercise can be used. These methods that can function as important stress relievers.

Another very important factor in this case is sleep. **Sleep deprivation can definitely lower one's libido**. Very little to no sleep can result to stress, which may directly affect the libido of a person. That radically reduces testosterone production and in return lowers down the libido level.

With this, it can be concluded that in order to achieve higher libido levels, it is necessary to increase our testosterone production in men as well as have proper blood circulation in both genders.

Chapter 3: Products that Increase Your Libido

There are many products that have been proven to increase the libido. Whether it is food or other items, take advantage of this list to really increase your libido. Some may be rare, but most can be found in your home pantry and the local stores nearby. Get ready to take down some notes.

Brazil Nut

A study from the University of Padua in Italy revealed that diets low in selenium may be one of the causes of male sterility. Selenium prevents oxidation (damage) of the sperm, which increases your chances of having healthy soldiers and better libido level.

Chocolate

Chocolates contain a substance called Phenylethylamine. Phenylethylamine is believed by many to be somewhat similar to a "Love Potion", as it can produce the feeling of being in love. Moreover, dark chocolate can also improve the blood circulation, increase blood flow in the brain, and prevents fatigue. Now, you know why chocolates are great aphrodisiacs.

Oysters

Another type of food that can increase libido would be oysters. Oysters were one of those foods that are labeled as aphrodisiacs. Some even call it a "Love Drug" and they do so for a good reason. Oysters can help in improving dopamine levels. Dopamine levels boost libido for both men and women.

In addition, oysters are also very in Zinc which is important in producing healthy sperms and for testosterone production.

Eggs and Chicken Meat

Feeling all too tired to have sex? It might be caused by mild anemia, which is quite common especially for women. Studies even show that mild anemia may just be the culprit behind fatigue as well as low sex drive. Eggs and chicken meat might help solve all of that. Eggs and chicken meat are great sources of iron. Eggs are rich in Vitamins B5 and B6. Such vitamins can fight off stress while also balancing the hormonal levels in the body. Aside from eggs and chicken meat, you can also rely on liver, dark turkey meat, and spinach. Those are also rich in iron.

Honey

Honey is such a simple food that many think of it a potent libido enhancer, but it actually is. Remember how after a wedding, a couple would go and get some honeymoon leave? Well, that rooted from our humble honey. Honeymoon came to be because before, to catch up, pairs of ancient Persia drank mead every day for the first month after marriage (the month of honey, or as we know, the "honeymoon").

Honey is rich in B vitamins, which are necessary to make testosterone and fructose. This makes you stronger and steadily releases energy. Rolling over and falling asleep will not be an option with honey in the picture.

Watermelon

What?! Not watermelon, too!!! Well, yes, it does even watermelon can help boost your libido. Though 92% of watermelon is basically water, the rest of it is actually rich in phytonutrient citrulline. The phytonutrient citrulline can be converted to arginine in the body. Arginine is an amino acid that helps in relaxing the blood vessels, especially around the erectile tissue. Scientists from Texas have shown that eating watermelon can have similar effects to those of the "miraculous" blue pill Viagra and the best part is that watermelon is healthy. You will need to pay attention to the specific season in which you are able to purchase watermelons, though as they do not come around every day.

Vanilla Ice Cream

Vanilla, are not used in everything from desserts to air fresheners, for nothing. According to the Foundation for Research and Treatment of Smell and Taste of Chicago (USA), vanilla may increase the blood flow in the penile area. For an extra oomph of sexuality, add vanilla scented candles to the atmosphere. If you are a female, you can purchase vanilla bean lotion or vanilla bean butter. Apply it after your showers for a "pick-me-up, cowboy" mode in the bedroom.

Ginger

A study was published in the journal, *"Phytomedicine"*. In this study, male rats which were given ginger experienced an increase in testicular weight. It is believed that ginger may have a similar effect of "swelling" in the testosterone human.

Pumpkin Seeds

Pumpkin seeds have a lot of zinc, a key nutrient for sexuality and fertility. A Dutch study found that supplements of folic acid and zinc increases sperm count by 74% in men with fertility problems. Pumpkin seeds can be purchased from any grocery store that carries items like sunflower seeds. They are typically found in the same aisle. Pumpkin seeds also come in a variety of flavors.

Popcorn

This classic movie food partner has the highest levels of plant arginine, which is the main component of semen. Numerous studies have demonstrated the importance of arginine for sperm count, quality, and mobility. So prepare a good portion and press play. Movie nights will never be the same again as you can make them intimate with popcorn, your libido will be soaring and so will your partner's. Have fun some poppin' fun!

Chili

We all know that spicy food accelerates the heart. Capsaicin, the compound that makes chili pique, also triggers the brain to release endorphins, which can make you feel great. Chili also improves the nervous system, which favors the excitation. Best to have a very "spicy" relationship, right?

Banana

Banana also helps in boosting sex drive. Whether it is dehydrated banana chips, or the fresh fruit, you can utilize this as a natural aphrodisiac. They will increase your libido merely by eating them.

Blueberry

According to studies made in the University of Texas (USA), insufficient amounts of vitamin C can cause sperm cells lose mobility. Blueberries are loaded with vitamin C for your sperms to swim like Michael Phelps.

Almonds

These nuts are packed with essential fats that regulate prostaglandins, vital for the production of sex hormones. Also contain vitamin E, which helps to make a stronger thanks to its antioxidant sperm.

Sirloin Steak

A study published in *"The Journal of Fertility and Sterility"* revealed that the sirloin, which contains large amounts of L-carnitine, significantly improved the quality of sperm in a group of men with fertility problems. It seems that the higher the level of L-carnitine is, the better the count and sperm motility are. Now, get up and go get some meat. You will not regret it. Who would turn down a nice juicy steak, then a romp in the bedroom?

Gambas

These marine animals contain large amounts of zinc, which improves libido and sperm production. They also have calcium and magnesium, necessary for muscle contraction that helps regulate sexual impulse, sperm count, and fertility. And the thing does not end there: they contain an ocean of phenylalanine, an amino acid that helps regulate mood and improve sexual appetite. This offers so many benefits to your sex life one might think it to be illegal. Luckily, it isn't and you can partake of this tasty marine animal and fill your tummy and your sex life.

Cucumber

Leaving aside the jokes, a study by the Foundation for Research and Treatment of Smell and Taste of Chicago (USA) found that one of the scents that trigger more arousal in women is, believe it or not, cucumber. Make a tasty appetizer combining chopped cucumber, mint leaves, and yogurt and you're on for a lovely night in bed.

Granada

This helps to prevent erectile dysfunction. Scientists believe that this is due to the potent antioxidant juice Granada, which prevents free radicals from creating chaos in your manhood. So take a cup if you want to get on morality.

Sesame Seeds

The size of these little seeds not does do justice to the Herculean strength they have in terms of being nutritious. In ancient Greek, brides received sesame cakes as a symbol for fruitfulness (which can be broadly interpreted as "luck in bed"). Sesame seeds contain lots of selenium and zinc. They are also rich in calcium, magnesium, vitamin E, and essential fats - all nutrients that are good for the libido.

Asparagus

Asparagus is rich in potassium and calcium, which helps hormone production while also increasing energy levels. They are also rich in vitamin E, which improves blood flow to the genitals.

Nata

No, it's not a typo. In moderation, nata is a great source of calcium, needed to improve muscle contraction associated with erection. It is also a good source of protein, which is found in high levels in sperm. Moreover, it is a supreme pleasure, which will add fun to the matter.

Peanut

This nut helps you maintain healthy vascular system, which ensures adequate blood flow to the trophy room. Peanuts are rich in Omega-3 fatty acids, which reduce cholesterol that clogs arteries and thus, decrease the risk of heart.

Spinach

If you eat this raw, this versatile vegetable is one of the few that contain coenzyme Q10. A study from *"The Journal of Fertility and Sterility"* found that coenzyme Q10 can help improve sperm movement, which is good news for those who need aid. The spinach also contains lots of iron, fighting infertility, according to a study by Harvard University (USA). Now you know why Popeye is so strong when eating his can of spinach.

Garlic

Garlic contains a potent ingredient called allicin, which increases blood flow and libido. But do not forget to take candy for your breath or you are going to get sent home early. Garlic is not just for those who love Italian food, but for those who love to have a healthy sex life.

Truffle

Truffles are on this list due to its intense aroma, a substance called alpha-androstenol, which mimics the smell of pheromones. These are hormones that trigger physical attraction. Serve breakfast gratin on scrambled eggs in bed, but be prepared to not leave until lunchtime, if you know what I mean.

Tomato

Tomatoes are known as the "love apples". This reputation is based on the tomato's color and touch. But more to that, tomatoes actually have high contents of beta-carotene, which your body converts into vitamin A. Vitamin A is vital in maintaining good sexual health. Vitamin A also plays an important role in the production of testosterone. So, gentlemen, if you are looking for something that is proven to work and is cheap, as well as natural - simply eat tomatoes. Tomatoes are great on sandwiches or even on your partner.

Tuna

This fish is rich in vitamin B3, which has an effect of dilating blood vessels. This in turn will help in improving your sex life. You may have enhanced orgasms, increased sensation of touch, and more powerful erections. So, make sure you have this on the menu in important dates.

Celery

The Romans used celery as an aphrodisiac. It contains lots of pheromones called androstenone and androstenol, which is believed to attract women. In addition, chewing celery can clean the teeth, another great point to impress your love.

Causes of a Low Libido and Lifestyle Changes

A low libido can be caused by a number of factors, including stress, lack of exercise, an unhealthy diet, certain medications, and hormones. Antidepressants can also decrease your libido and with these involved, libido is even harder to spur back.

A low libido can affect your marriage, since sex plays a major role in any good relationship. Sure, some people can just go and grab a Viagra for a more intensified love play, but for many people it can be very expensive. Instead of spending money on prescription drugs, why not increase your libido naturally with herbs and supplements, eating food right, and exercising? There are simple and inexpensive methods to increase libido without having to spend a large sum of money on commercial remedies.

Chapter 4: Pregnancy, the Libido Killer

Pregnancy is an important time of change - both physically and emotionally. The constant evolution of the body and the roller coaster of emotions during those nine months may confound any woman, especially those who are unable to control their emotions. The belly grows in size and becomes rounded in shape, the breasts grow, as well as its sensitivity and mood swings are varying depending on the day without a specific reason at all. How do these changes affect the libido of women?

Sexual Desire During Pregnancy

The sexual life of the couple may be affected during the duration of pregnancy. While each and every woman is facing body changes differently, it is true that sex will still be affected in most cases - one form or another.

There are women whose sexual desire disappear completely during pregnancy. Some women in their first trimester may begin to suffer nausea and other discomforts that hormonal change slaps on their body. This makes them more engaged in "fighting off" the bad feelings of inconvenience. This makes them "unconcerned" about sex life.

Their sexual desire may also be affected by the fears and insecurities brought about by their current looks and situation. The fear of harming the baby or cause miscarriage lowers sex drive considerably. It also occurs in many cases that pregnant women feel less attractive because their body has transformed and therefore less desired by their partner.

By contrast, there are other women who experience an exaggerated increase sexual desire, even during pregnancy, especially in the second trimester. Their increased hormone levels resulted in cases of increased vaginal lubrication, hypersensitive breasts, and a smoother blood circulation in the pelvic area. All this can make women feel more energized for sex.

Keeping the Passion Alive During Pregnancy

As every woman is different, two situations can occur related to a woman's sexual desire - sexual desire increases or disappears altogether. Not to worry though. Always keep in mind that this is just a temporary situation.

Nevertheless, to ensure that libido is maintained at acceptable levels the aid and support of the partner would be required. Though the future father may be suffering from the loss of sexual desire, pregnancy is not the time to be selfish. Your pregnant partner needs you and you can both support each other while going through the pregnancy stage.

The truth is that sex during pregnancy is entirely desirable, as long as both partners want it. However, there are special cases when sex is not advisable to keep. Such cases would include having a history of pre-term delivery and placenta previa or bleeding, among others.

If there are doubts about whether or not you can have sex, you must seek medical care immediately for resolution and perform ongoing tests to know at all times that the pregnancy develops correctly.

Here is a timeline to help identify a woman's changing libido during pregnancy:

Changes during the first trimester of pregnancy

There may be decreased libido in this trimester because of the **changes that occur in pregnancy** like fatigue, nausea, and vomiting. This is typically referred to as *morning sickness*. Morning sickness can last anywhere from 1 to 3 months in the first trimester. Some women will experience morning sickness throughout their entire pregnancy due to high hcg levels.

There is also an **increased sensitivity and breast tenderness** in some women, which may lead them to become more agitated and upset. This is due to the fact that their breasts are developing for the arrival of the baby as well as to accommodate the baby's needs.

There may also be a **level of anxiety for fear of interrupting the pregnancy**. This is not just a fear that women experience. Many fathers have also expressed their fear of harming their unborn child due to the sex activities they do. If you feel unsure if you are able to have sex safely, speak with your doctor.

Changes During the Second Trimester

During the second quarter the situation changes considerably since many of the fears and the initial discomfort may have already disappeared. This stage is similar to the regular pre-pregnancy stage. During this time, relationships may be more satisfying because of the physiological changes that occur. Among them these changes include **increased**

congestion of the tissues surrounding the vagina, as well as **increased lubrication**, which can increase arousal.

However, at this trimester, it is time to **adjust to new positions**, because as the uterus increases in size, certain positions may be uncomfortable for the pregnant partner. One of the positions that can be comfortable for the woman would be the *"Woman on Top"* position since this position allows better control of the weight, the degree of penetration, and intensity of sex. If the man is on top, he must ensure that he does not load all his weight on the abdomen of his lady love. That said, it is still advised that the missionary position be avoided completely for safety. Another position or technique that most couple also use is the one where the woman is on her hands and knees to ensure no pressure is put on the abdomen of the woman.

Changes During the Third Trimester

This is the most crucial trimester of all. The belly has not increased considerably and the baby nears his or her full term. In this light, though many doctors would advise to abstain from sex completely, there are still cases when you can have sex sparingly. In light with that, there are some things that you need to consider.

Talk with your partner regarding the best sex position for her. What position is she most comfortable with? Remember, she is already bearing a full grown baby inside her and doing sex will actually burden her a little more, but if she wants to have sex, too, better talk it out with her so sex can still be enjoyable.

At this point, the **anxiety level of both partners may be at its peak** due to the impending birth of the baby. This can be applied for both genders so be sure to consider this as well before requesting for sex.

Aside from those mentioned, the **semen secreted at orgasm may also produce mild contractions and help the onset of labor**. Should the woman have any complication during the pregnancy, the doctor may ask that the couple does not have sex during this trimester. On the other hand, if the woman is ready to give birth the doctor may encourage the couple to have sex to onset labor.

Chapter 5: Positivity

Have a **positive mental attitude** and **keep your stress levels low**. If you feel good and trust yourself, you will be more sexually attractive to your partner. Prolonged stress can lead to decreased interest in sex. People working in stressful jobs or who have a long commute to work (we all know how it can be stressful traffic) often have poor sex drives.

Men and women react differently to stressful situations manner. For men, sex is often a stressful release of energy while for women, stress blocks sex in their minds. Sex is plainly not their solution for stress. If that is the case, sex will not be enjoyed by both partners. As such, it would be better to delay sex so stress can be resolved. Once everything is stress free, you and your partner can simply go for sex all day long and still be assured that both of you will love the experience.

Libido: Consuming the Right Natural Supplements and Food

Libido can also be enhanced with the use of natural supplements not only for fighting stress, but also for solving factors that may hurt your libido. For instance, natural supplements can help increase blood flow and sometimes help combat vaginal dryness. Some natural supplements that can increase libido include vitamin E, zinc, vitamin C, vitamin B6, and vitamin B complex. These nutrients can help men increase your sperm count, help enhance the function of the prostate gland, increase testosterone production, and create a healthier nervous system.

Some foods that may increase the libido include celery, raw oysters, bananas, avocados, peaches, strawberries, eggs, liver, figs, garlic, pumpkin, and chocolate. Certain foods and natural supplements like these can add lots of nutrients and minerals to your diet, but is unlikely to have an impact on your behavior and sexual performance, these include would include the following:

(1) A **healthy, nutrient-supported proteins, limiting saturated fat and a variety of fruits and vegetables** diet (note that saturated fat can clog your arteries and prevent blood flow to your genitals);

(2) Intake of **vitamins and omega 3 and 6** to address the deficiencies in your diet;

(3) **Regular exercise** endurance and strength; and

(4) Achieve and maintain a **healthy body fat percentage**

You can also **alleviate oxidative stress with NAC (acetyl cysteine) and other antioxidants**. NAC is a precursor of glutathione. Glutathione is the *"mother of all antioxidants."* Antioxidants help dilate blood vessels, causing efficient blood flow as well as aid in resolving erectile dysfunction.

With the ingestion of three capsules (600 mg each) of NAC per day, there is also an observable increase in natural good humor and an increasing standard of basic robustness that we all use to calculate our "natural" age. More NAC will definitely make you feel younger.

Besides feeling better and younger by increasing the intake of NAC, a natural boost libido is undeniable. Other strong antioxidants that can help in increasing libido would include coffee, cranberries, walnuts, and green tea.

Libido: Setting Up the Right Environment

The environment can also play a great part in setting up the mood and heightening the libido. There are certain stimulants that turn yours or your partner's libido, on and off.

To avoid ruining the mood, **remove the certain items from your bedroom**. Remove the pictures of your parents or your children, as there are people who feel awkward with such pictures. They feel like being watched and this is a major turn off. Any mess would also have the same libido-decreasing effect. This includes piles of papers, books, and work-related documents.

To help put the environment on fire (figuratively, of course), **choose soft lighting** that can set the mood. Soft lighting may be in the form of scented candles, low voltage bulbs, or colored lights giving off a romantic vibe.

Get some fresh air in through the window and use some incense, oils or scents that smell rich. Use soft aromas, wear your best perfume, but be sure it is not too strong so as not to put the sexual desire off.

Coffee and chocolate are good to eat before sex. Both are considered aphrodisiacs because they produce positive moods, release endorphins, energize, and increase body resistance.

Wine and other alcoholic beverages can help you relax, but because alcohol is a natural depressant, sometimes it makes some people feel depressed or wanting to sleep. Alcohol and sexual performance does not match well with some men.

Sexual role-playing can spark magic for you and your partner. Sexual desire tends to be associated with different situations for different people. No need to recreate every detail of those situations though. with a little imagination, improvisation, and interpretation of characters, you can incorporate one or two key elements of the situation you want to recreate. These small elements can raise your sexual desire level. Sometimes, it's best to start with an approach that you understand more if you're new to role-playing games with your partner. Often with just a hint of something, some people get excited, and this may be sufficient enough to raise the desire and attraction.

Seek help from a sex therapist if necessary. If you are experiencing sexual problems like desire, initiation, or less enjoyment of sex, considering it as something psychological. If this is your case, seek professional help. Sex therapists treat cases of impotence or loss of sexual appetite that can result from a hidden depression. Sex therapists also provide talks to individuals and couples and often provide them tasks and activities to help revive normal levels of sexual function.

For example, sex therapists can encourage you to explore different ways of being close to each other without having intercourse. This will help rebuild confidence, a sense of mutual acceptance, and not to judge on the bed. The main idea of these tasks is to eliminate the association of sex with stress, pressure, and disappointment. These tasks also help you to re-associate sex with fun, mutual acceptance, exploration, and pleasuring.

Be patient. If your partner is being treated for loss of interest and enjoyment of sex or problems regarding sexual performance, be patient and realize that treatment can take many months or more to be effective.

If you're starting to date someone who has these problems, you have no obligation to go out with them because we all have the right to find a partner who can sexually satisfy us. You can end the relationship because they are not sexually compatible with you or for any other reason. Alternatively, you can try to be patient, but if you think it will not work, you better tell immediately and not after a long time when it is most painful for the other person.

Understand the role of testosterone and its relation to sexual behavior in the long-term for both men and women. Based on studies and trials, the libido of a woman and interest to initiate sex responds to testosterone supplements. These supplements have been tested in Europe, but are still undergoing trials in the United States. On the other hand, men usually receive testosterone supplements from their doctors to treat low testosterone levels, increase libido, and enhance sexual performance. The natural production of testosterone in men and women tends to decline with age and this natural decline can be accelerated by smoking, drinking, having excess body fat, and the likes.

The **natural levels of testosterone in men increases in the mornings**, so if you and your partner have sexual problems or if your man's interest has decreased lately, try having sex in the morning for an extra sex oomph.

Performs feats of strength and endurance, which will increase your testosterone levels while also helping you increase your energy levels. Some push-ups, weight lifting, or squats can help rebuild muscle and make your testosterone production increase. Often an increase in testosterone and sexual behavior can be noticed immediately after a workout. Many couples even exercise together, as this can serve as their sexual stimulant. Moreover, when combined with proper diet, this can help remove excess body fat, which may cause low testosterone level.

Chapter 6: Acceptance is the Key

You need to remember that no human is perfect. No matter how much you would want your partner or yourself to have high libido 100% of the time, it will just not happen. You have to accept the fact that there would be fluctuations in the libido level of you and your partner and this is due to many reasons.

This may be **due to age-related changes and the progression of our development period**. If you are a man, you're probably not as interested in sex as you were when you were just 18 years old. If you are a woman your current level of interest may increase when you turn 30 and in both genders a decline can be expected when you turn 60.

Sometimes **radical changes in sexual behavior may occur because of varying hormone levels**. This is perfectly normal and may possibly be temporary. So, do not stress yourself out. Remember, stress is also a contributing factor. Stay calm and collected.

For instance, women may experience an increase in sexual behavior during ovulation, menstruation, and unexpectedly while pregnant. Moreover, women may experience a decrease in their libido in the first few months after giving birth, while breastfeeding and after menopause. All of these cases are due to their fluctuating hormonal changes. Some women experience a decrease in libido after starting birth control treatment since birth control treatments trick the body into thinking that women are pregnant.

It is important to be patient with women who have just given birth. Men would have to understand that it will take approximately 3 or 4 months to raise their sexual appetite back because their bodies have suffered from the trauma of giving birth to a baby and their bodies are still adjusting to the stabilization of their hormone levels.

If you are a woman whose libido has dropped by more than a couple of months, this may represent a problem from your perspective. If this decline is not due to intake of birth control pills, giving birth or early menopause, seek professional help to rule out any abnormalities.

Warnings to Keep in Mind

Never use a prescription medication which is not prescribed to you by your doctor. Even if the medication promises to increase your sexual performance if it was not prescribed to you by your doctor it may just be dangerous for you. Such medications may bring about unwanted side effects or they may be contraindicated to the medications that you are currently taking.

Do not expect aphrodisiacs to work magically. Many natural aphrodisiacs are simply diuretics, which mean you will urinate more frequently such as coffee. Diuretics may be sexual stimulants and great means for increasing your desire of sex, but do not expect a dramatic change in your sexual behavior.

Illegal steroids can increase your libido, but at a very high cost. They can cause you long-term health issues, especially to your heart as well as irreversible changes to your body. There are many legal and safe supplements related to increased strength and steroid-like results without risking any permanent damage.

Talk to your doctor about **medications that may be suppressing your libido.** A variety of medications can interfere with your libido and your sexual performance. The benefits of some medicines like anti-depressants may interfere with your sex life. The decision to reduce the dose or stop medication intake can only be recommended by your doctor. Discuss your questions with your doctor so he or she will know what to do.

Beware of herbal blends that promise to increase your libido. Some can cause uncomfortable erections that can last for hours, increase your heart rate, and make your heart beat fast. Talk to your doctor before taking any drug or herb to see if it is safe to try.

The first step to increase your libido is **stop using drugs and alcohol**. If you smoke marijuana, hooked to drinking alcohol, or use drugs like amphetamines, cocaine, or heroin, you may just be accelerating the process of a declining sexual appetite and lack of libido. All these substances suppress testosterone production. For example, an alcoholic beverage may suppress the production of testosterone and stops the possibility of developing muscle mass per 24 hours.

Changing these habits and then working on the next steps we have seen in the article can increase your libido so enjoy your sexual life again.

Conclusion

Thank you again for downloading this book!

I hope this book was able to help you increase you and/or your partner's libido.

The next step is well… after reading this book, you should get the picture…

Finally, if you enjoyed this book, please take the time to share your thoughts and post a review on Amazon. It'd be greatly appreciated!

Thank you and good luck!

www.ingramcontent.com/pod-product-compliance
Lightning Source LLC
Chambersburg PA
CBHW070522290526
45790CB00003B/1272